The Prostate
illustrated

in 10 points

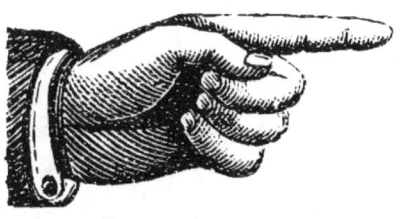

for the patients

.

Text and illustrations: Dr Bertrand Vayleux

TABLE OF CONTENTS

The Prostate illustrated

TABLE OF CONTENTS

The Prostate illustrated

ISBN: 1533218838
ISBN-13: 9781533218834

WARNING

THIS DOCUMENT IS INTENDED FOR PATIENTS AND THEIR FAMILIES.

THE DISCLOSURES IN THESE CHAPTERS ARE LIKELY TO BE EXCEEDED IN THE COMING YEARS.

THIS DOCUMENT DOES NOT REPLACE A CONSULTATION WITH A UROLOGIST BUT ON THE CONTRARY IT OPENS THE WAY FOR YOU.

The Prostate illustrated

1 - THE PROSTATE

What is the prostate?

It's a little gland usually the size of a chestnut, made of muscular cells and glandular tissue.

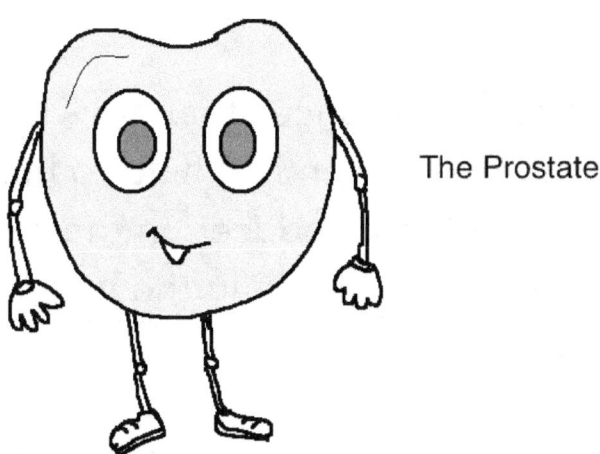

The Prostate

It is composed of two parts; the central zone, that as patients age in their 50's, can become responsible for certain urinary tract disorders. This is what is called **benign prostatic hyperplasia (BPH).**

The second part, peripheral, is where most often prostate cancer develops, also called **prostatic adenocarcinoma**.

The entire gland is covered with a thin shell, the prostatic capsule.

The Prostate participates only in **reproductive function.**

It produces substances that are components of the seminal fluid to help sperm (themselves produced in the testicles) to keep their vitality once in the vagina and the uterus.

It has no role in urinary function, rather it just acts as a troublemakers.

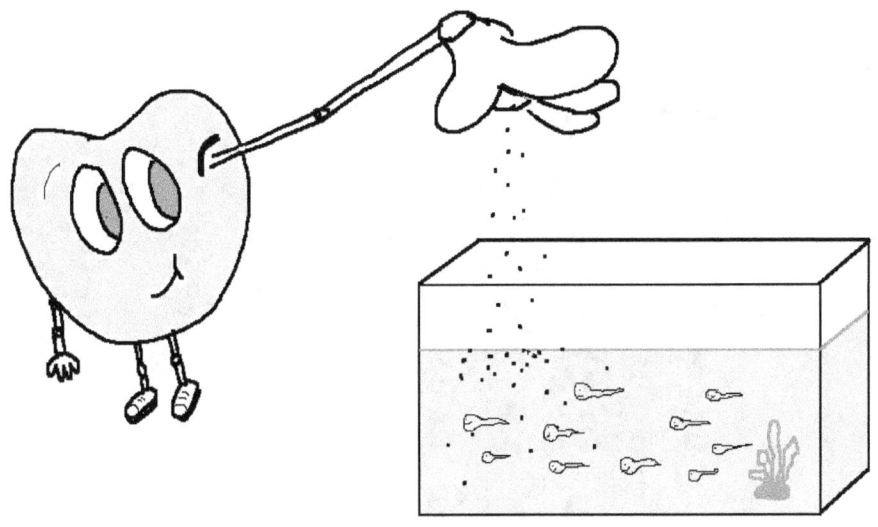

The prostate ensure sperm viability

Where is the prostate?

It is located in the pelvis, under the bladder and in front of the rectum. The urinary channel through the urethra is like an apple core.

Two small reservoirs, seminal vesicles, are connected towards the back. They contain seminal fluid.

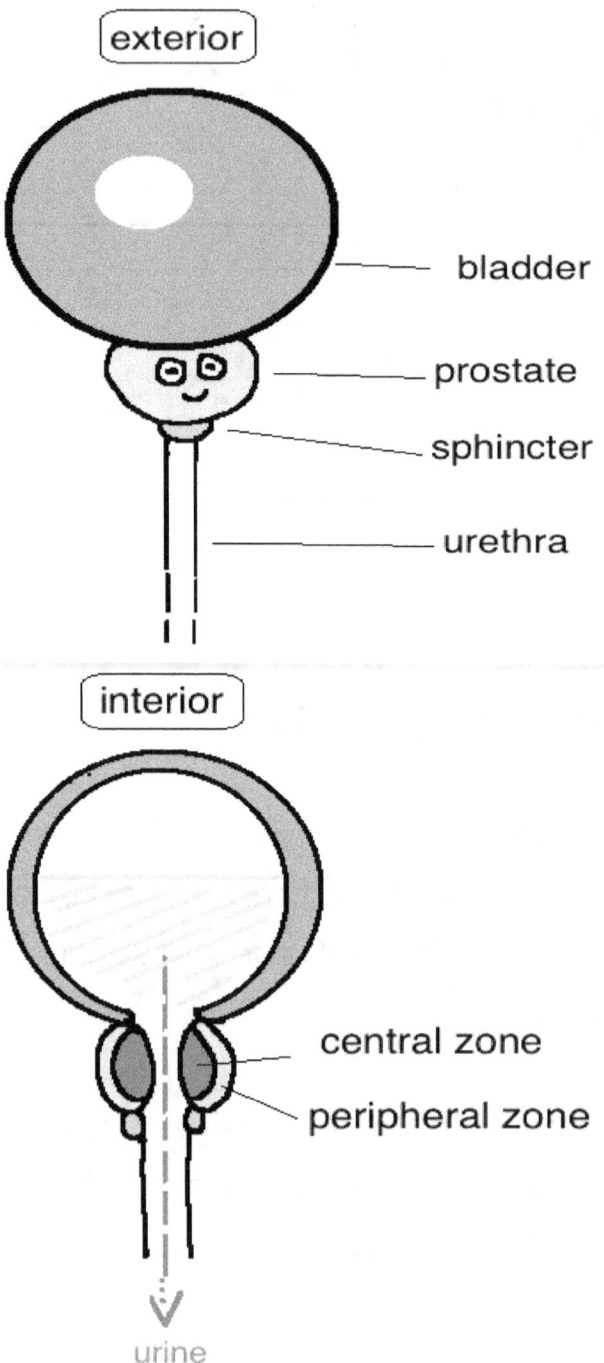

exterior

bladder

prostate

sphincter

urethra

interior

central zone

peripheral zone

urine

2 - THE PSA

Prostate marker

The Prostate Specific Antigen (PSA) originates only in the prostate. It is produced by normal prostate cells, and levels can increase (10 times) with cancerous prostate cells. The PSA is measured in a **blood test**.

This analysis is intended only to the **early diagnosis of prostate cancer**. It is prescribed from men in their 50's up to 75 years, or to 45 years olds if certain risk factors are met (see section on prostate cancer) according to European recommendations.

This PSA is not specific for prostate cancer

and levels **may be increased for various reasons**, such as urinary tract infections, most commonly prostate inflammation, pressure on the prostate, etc ...

The volume of the prostate, and the patient's age may be responsible for a progressive increase in the PSA.

So it is therefore difficult to draw conclusions on the health of the prostate with a single PSA test. Similarly, it is necessary to take into consideration the **overall context**, i.e. age, volume of the prostate, the presence of other diseases, etc ...

Two forms of PSA can be measured, total PSA and free PSA. This particular test is of greater interest when the rate is between 4 and 10, a grey area where the risk of prostate cancer is close to 30% (1). The report on the total free PSA is more reassuring above 0.25

(25%), or more worryingly below 0.15 (15%).

A PSA greater than 1.5 in 50 year olds or greater than 2.0 in 60 year olds is accompanied by a greater risk of developing prostate cancer. Annual monitoring of PSA levels is so important in these cases.

In contrast, with a lower rate of less than 1.0 in 60 year olds, the risk of dying from prostate cancer would drop to less than 2%.

AGE	PSA	
40-49	0 à 2.5	
50-59	0 à 3.5	*PSA threshold values (2)*
60-69	0 à 4.5	
70-79	0 à 6.5	

Some calculations are possible with the PSA, such as the doubling time of PSA, which may have be of interest in monitoring after treatment.

Other markers are under study but not in common use. PCA3 marker is recovered in the urine after prostatic massage. It would be particularly useful after a first series of negative prostate biopsies in the case of elevated PSA. A score over 35 would support a cancer. In France, this test costs around 300 euros.

And after 75 years...

After this age, it is not recommended to monitor PSA in the absence of **symptoms** suggestive of prostate cancer (new bone pain, fatigue, etc ..).

Prostate cancer most often evolves **slowly** over the years, at this age where the risk of having a different health problem increases with time.

Assuming that a man over 75 years old, who previously had a medical follow up, contracts prostate cancer, the symptoms can take years to arise, and in this case lead to a treatment that would usually reach or exceed the age of 77.8 years who is now the life expectancy for men in European country.

Medicines and PSA

In the often asked question: are there medications that can lower the PSA? The answer is yes, but is it desirable?

This would have interest if the prostate cancer risk decreases too. To date, there is no preventive treatment for this disease.

Finasteride and Dutasteride are two drugs prescribed for urinary disorders that originate from enlarged prostate. These two drugs lower the PSA to levels considered decreased by 30 to 50% in a few months.

While Dutasteride would decrease the risk of prostate cancer, at the same time it would be associated with more aggressive forms of cancer (3). Meanwhile, this drug isn't recommended in the prevention of this disease.

Other drugs would be associated with lower levels of PSA as aspirin, statins (against cholesterol), certain diuretics, etc ... without a positive effect on the prostate cancer being visible.

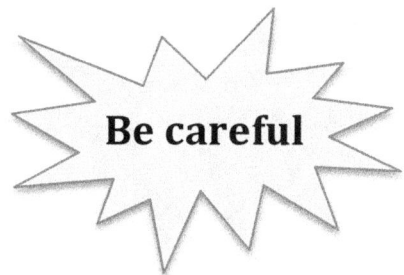

Be careful Herbal dietary supplements propose to lower the PSA. Beware, these products have often recieved no study or analysis and can even be dangerous depending on the doses used.

Advice Wait at least 6 to 8 weeks before dosing the PSA after prostate infection, retention of urine or after prostate biopsies.

The day of testing, avoid cycling or sexual intercourse (ejaculation).

Finally, it is advisable to use the same laboratory for analysis of any tests, because of the variability of dosing between machines.

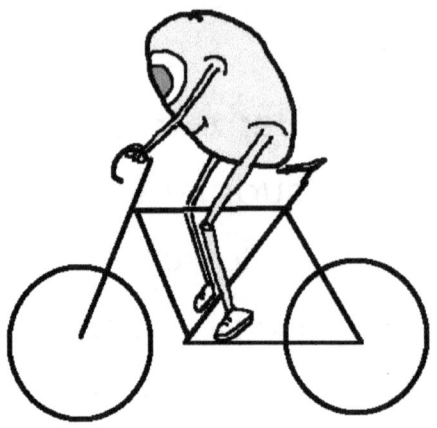

<u>Cycling and PSA</u>

The influence of cycling on the PSA is discussed. While on a purely theoretical level elevated PSA is explained on a practical level, several studies have shown no change in PSA levels before and after a bike race (4). However, avoid cycling on the day before undergoing a PSA assay.

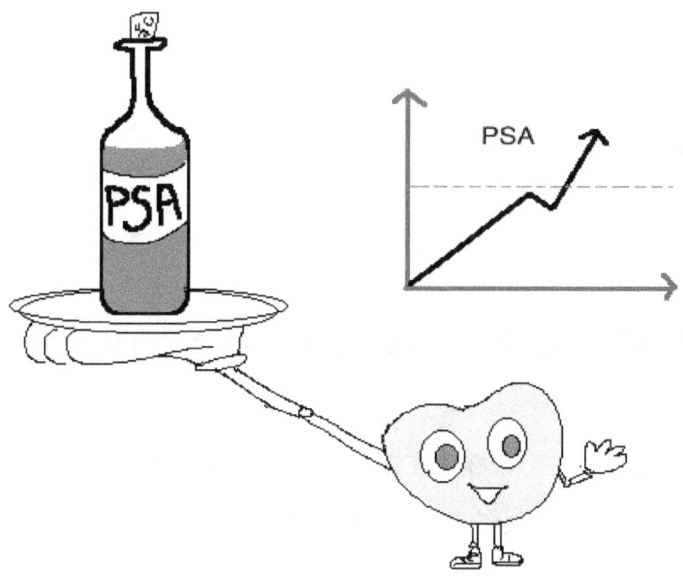

The PSA is produced by the prostate,
and this one increases in different circumstances

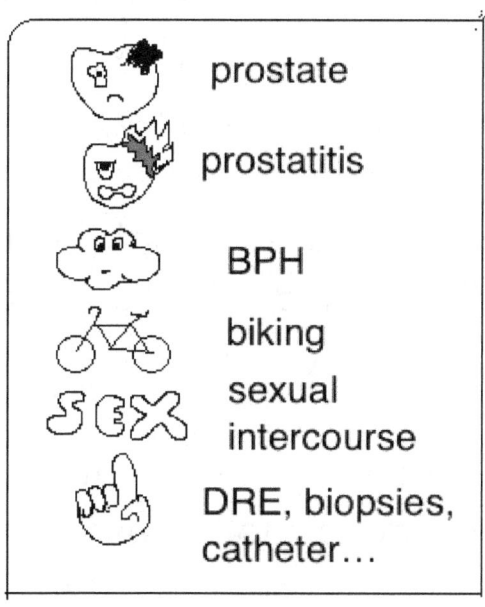

prostate

prostatitis

BPH

biking

sexual intercourse

DRE, biopsies, catheter…

3- DIGITAL RECTAL EXAMINATION

It's the dreaded moment. You are unable to escape it during your consultation with a Urologist.

Yet it is an essential examination since approximately 18% of cases, prostate cancer is detected by suspect prostate examination alone, whatever PSA level (5).

The doctor searches for information on the size of the gland, its consistency and sensitivity.

Digital rectal examination without abnormality does not mean there is no cancer, only one side of the prostate is accessible to the finger. The feeling of any abnormality is often accompanied by bad news.

So a suspicious touch means to complete a prostate biopsy.

This examination is also useful in prostatitis to confirm that the prostate is inflamed. The prostate is then unusually painful.

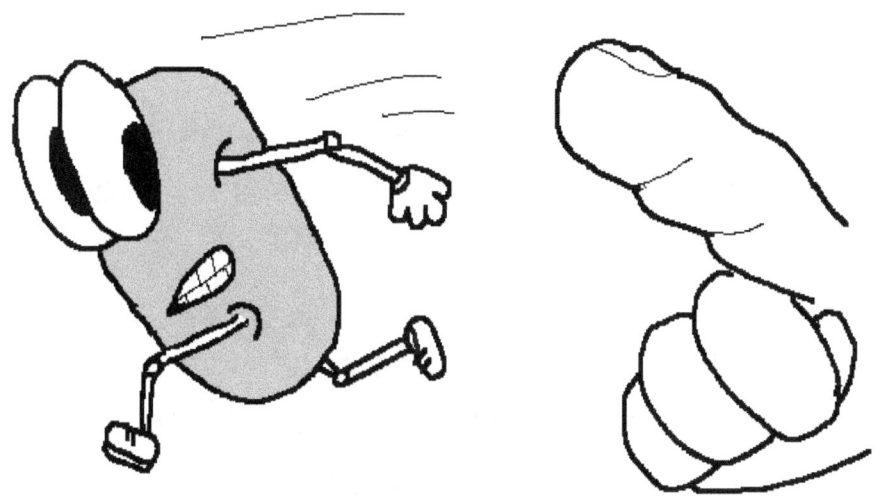

Digital rectal examination

4 – PROSTATE BIOPSY

The principle

This is the key exam of prostate cancer diagnosis.

It is proposed when repeated abnormal PSA levels are measured or after a suspectful prostate examination.

Analysis of tissue samples for the presence of cancer cells, and their characteristics.

This diagnostic test can be performed under local anesthesia with infiltration of a product near the prostate, or the patient may be completely asleep with general anesthesia.

A tracking takes place using a special ultrasound probe, slightly bigger than an index finger, introduced through the anus. Usually, a urine analysis is realized a few days before.   A dozen samples will be taken for a period of just 5 minutes.

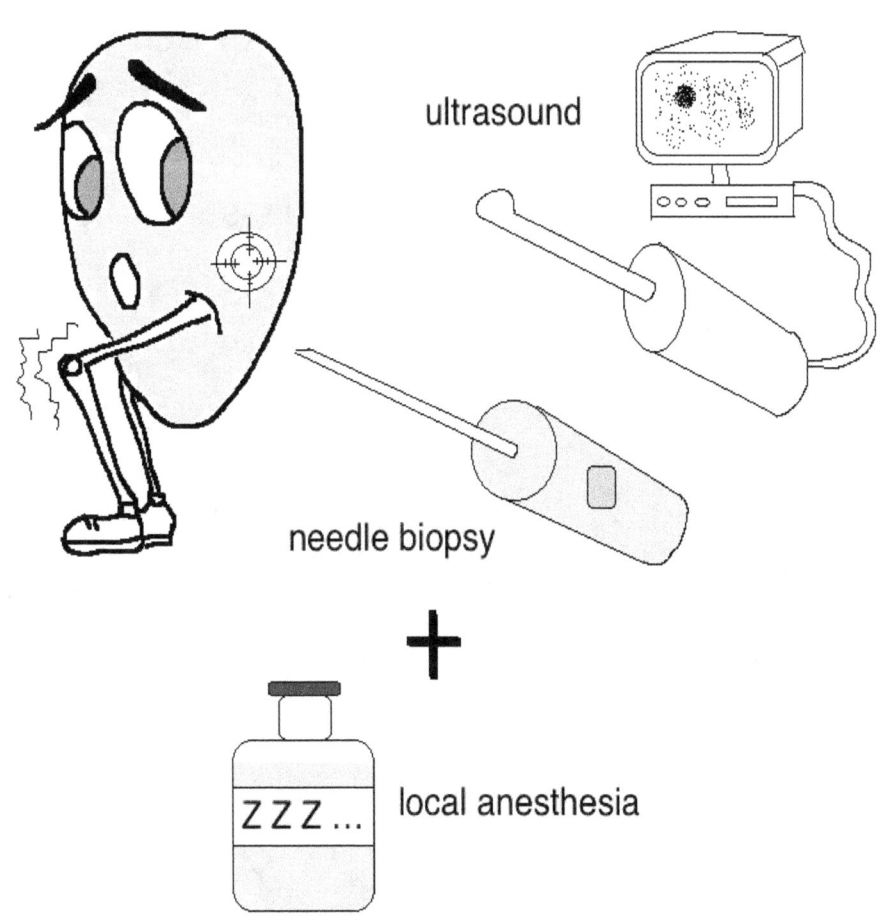

ultrasound

needle biopsy

local anesthesia

Complications

A little **blood** in the urine, semen or stool often happens in the early days. Specific instructions are given to people under treatments that cause bleeding.

Urinary retention (blockage) can occur, especially in men with pre existing urinary disorders.

Finally, a prostate infection called **prostatitis** can occur in less than 5% of cases.

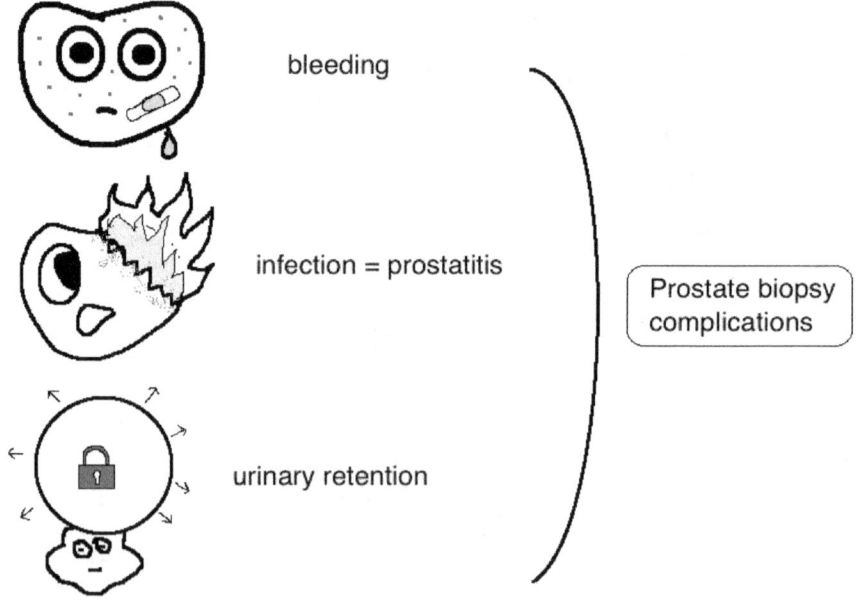

bleeding

infection = prostatitis

urinary retention

Prostate biopsy complications

The biopsy report

The presence of cancer cells is specified, their quantity by biopsy, and information on cancer cells aggressivity called the **Gleason Score**.

This Gleason Score has prognostic value, it helps to predict the evolution of the disease.

The most conventional forms of prostate cancer are Gleason 6 or 7. The most severe forms can go up to 10.

This score does not reflect the extent of the disease, this is the TNM (Tumor Nodes Metastasis) classification given by imaging studies (CT, MRI, etc.).

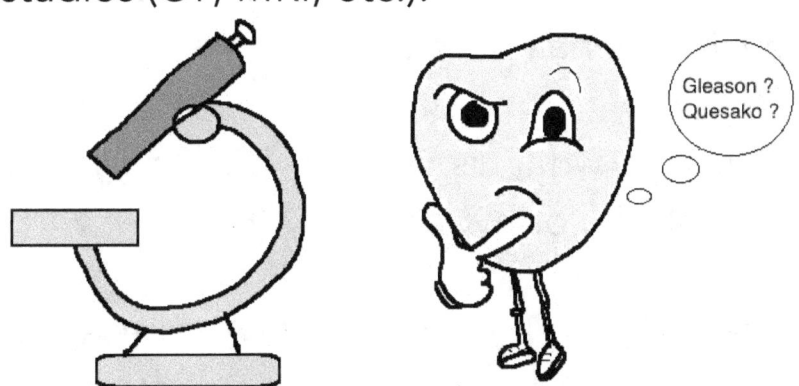

microscopic analysis

5 – THE BIG PROSTATE : BENIGN PROSTATE HYPERTROPHY

In general, the prostate enlarges over the age of fifty. 20 gr at 20 years old, it can reach more than 200 gr later.

However, there is no direct relationship between the size and urinary disorders. We find large prostates without problems and devilishly small prostates.

This is what is called benign prostatic hyperplasia, or hypertrophy (BPH).

Half of men over 60 and 80% of those over 80 years suffer from this problem (6).

Men with overweight (whose waist circumference exceeds 109 cm), are more at risk of having their prostate enlarged, and losing weight would improve this (7).

The central part of the prostate, which is in contact with the urinary tract, increases in volume and therefore reduces the size of the channel which crosses the urethra.

The prostate becomes an obstacle for the flow of urine and the upstream bladder can wear quickly.

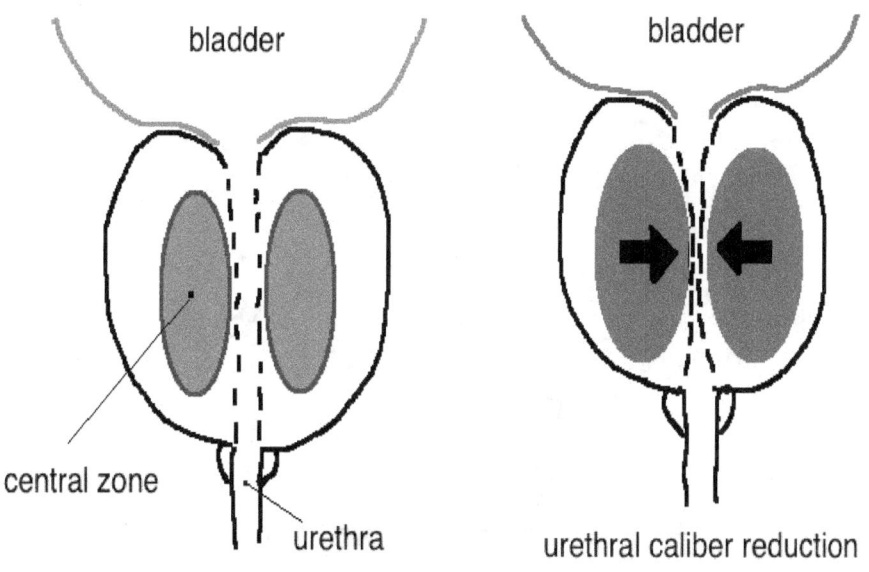

Urinary disorders

There are two categories of symptoms. The former are described as **obstructive**. For example, it can be observed the need to strain or push to initiate and maintain urination in order to more fully evacuate the bladder, with a decreased force of stream that comes dangerously close to the shoes, it can feel that the bladder does not empty completely, or a few straggling drops will remain to decorate the underwear.

in the moment

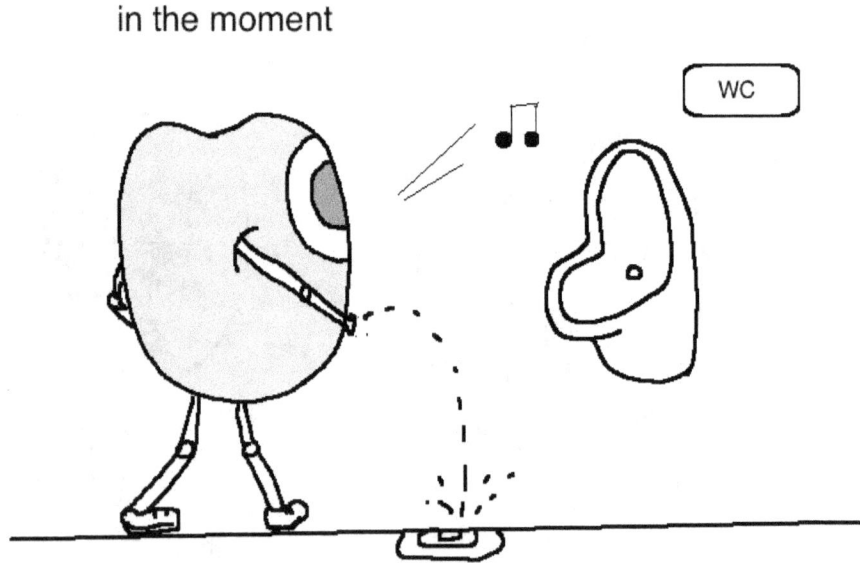

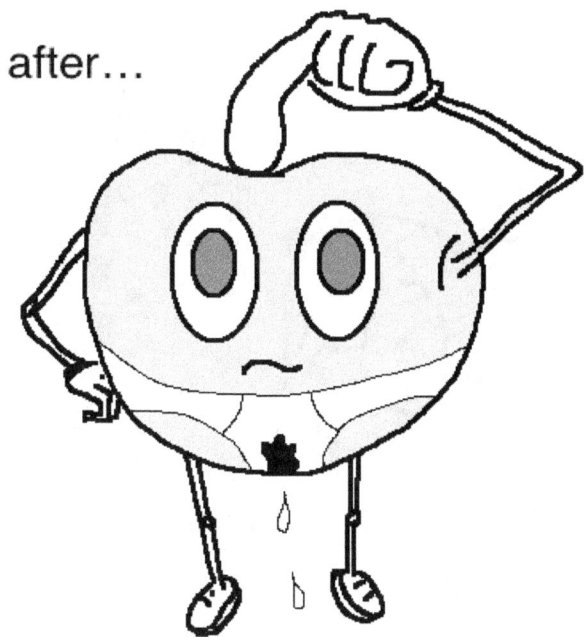

after…

Other symptoms are **irritative**. These are urgent or frequent desire to urinate, or the need to get up frequently at night to urinate small amounts.

nighttime urination

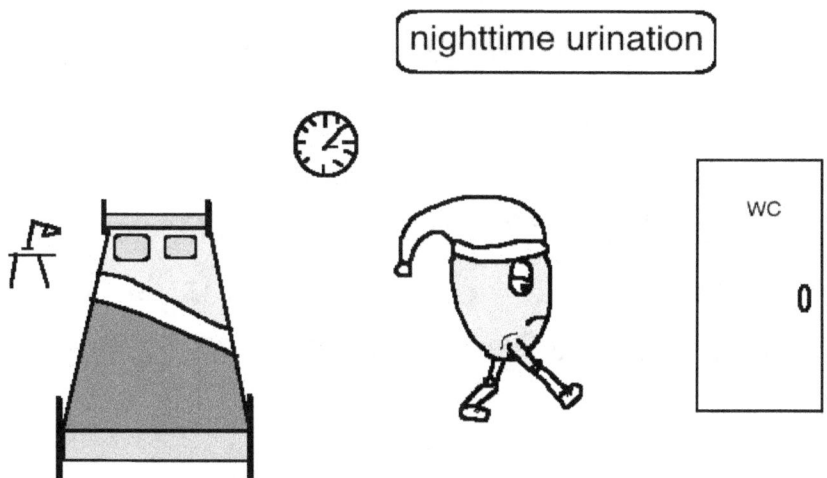

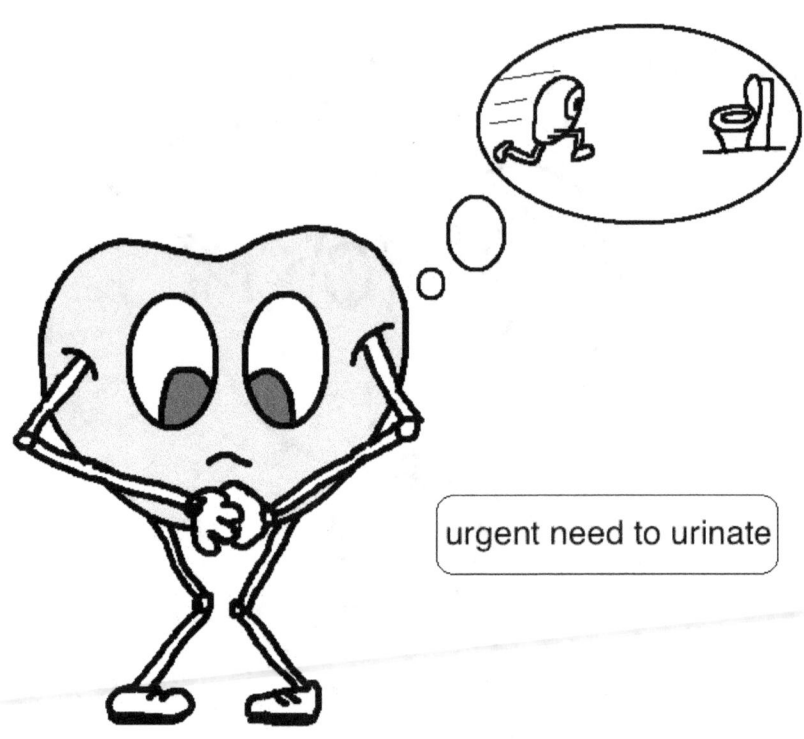

The prostate adenoma can give a mixture of all these urinary disorders.

In these situations, the bladder gradually thickens, then finally it exhaust itself with areas of weakness called diverticula.

Medical investigations

- PSA and digital rectal examination

- Uroflowmetry: urinary flow evaluation

- Bladder and prostate ultrasounds

- The symptom questionnaire

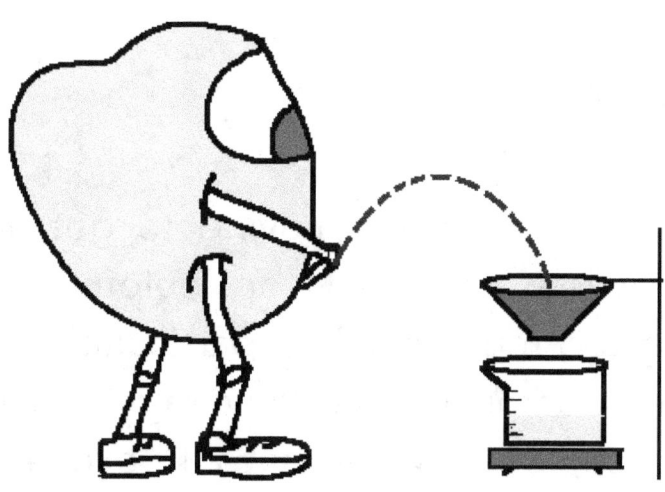

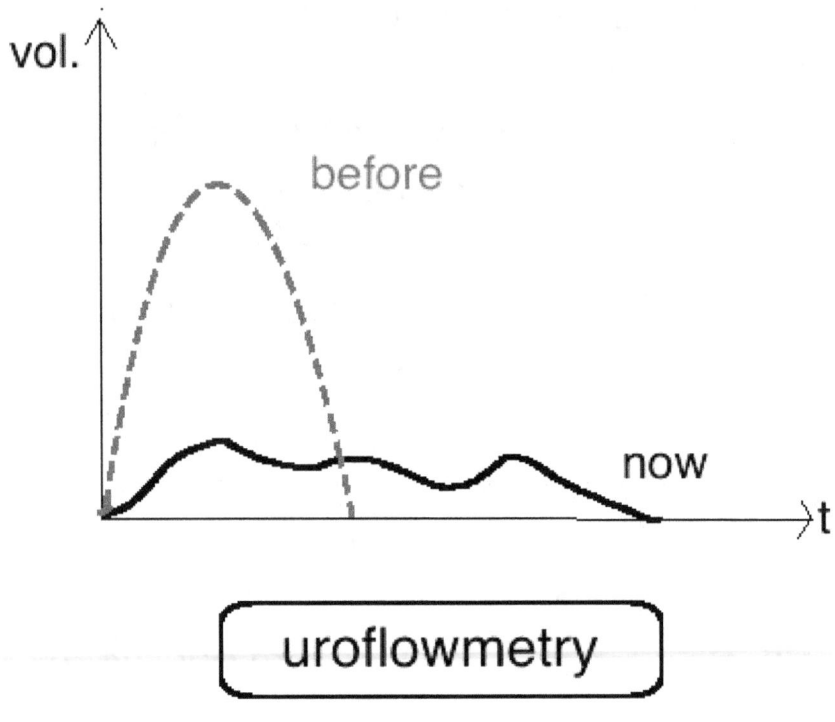

uroflowmetry

Advice

To avoid having to get up at night, a few tips may be helpful; avoid drinking too much alcohol, particularly in the evening, but also other beverages such as tea, coffee, white wine that all "excite" the bladder.

The treatments

○ <u>Mild urinary disorders:</u>

Phytotherapy (herbal and plant treatment), can be interesting due to their good tolerance.

As for the effects, they are modest, they are based on studies with lower levels of evidence, their effects differ from one laboratory to another, and the amount of active ingredient within the same brand (8).

Saw Palmetto (Serenoa repens) and the African plum tree (Pygeum africanum) are the best known and could help improve prostatic urinary disorders better than placebos.

Cucurbita pepo (Squash) contains linoleic acid. It is an antioxidant which would reduce BPH. It is often prescribe in association with the Saw palmetto. A study has shown that high intake may be toxic to the prostate (9).

Hypoxis Rooperi (African potato) is an antioxidant, it improves urine flow.

Secale Cereale (pollen) would decrease nighttime urination especially.

Urtica Dioica (Nettle), it's extract give a better urine flow and better bladder emptying.

Roystonea Regia (Royal Palm), studied in rats, the extract would reduce the size of the prostate.

- o <u>Moderate to severe urinary disorders:</u>

Drug treatment becomes necessary. The large family of "**alpha blockers**" will cause a relaxation in prostate and bladder neck level for better urine flow and better emptying of the bladder.

The common side effects include discomfort or dizziness associated with low blood pressure and **retrograde ejaculation**. This last point is often a source of anxiety for the patient, who once explained more readily accepts this type of unpleasantness. At the time of ejaculation, nothing comes out but sperm goes into the bladder.

For larger prostates, a second treatment may be associated with alpha blockers, either *Dutasteride* or *Finasteride*. Their goal is to reduce prostate volume. Slower than the first drug, its side effect of lowering the PSA levels artificially. It has not been concluded to date preventive effect on prostate cancer.

The side effects mostly relate sexuality with decreased libido, retrograde ejaculation and impotence.

○ <u>The surgery:</u>

When medications are not enough, a more radical treatment is necessary.

Endoscopic resection of prostate is a procedure through the urinary tract, under anesthesia, which winds up in the prostate, where the channel has a reduced caliber, scraping piece after piece into a lodge called cavity of resection.

Pieces of prostate removed are then sent for analysis. Duration: less than an one hour intervention, hospitalization for 3-4 days.

The risk of urinary incontinence is rare (1%), there's no erectile dysfunction but a final retrograde ejaculation.

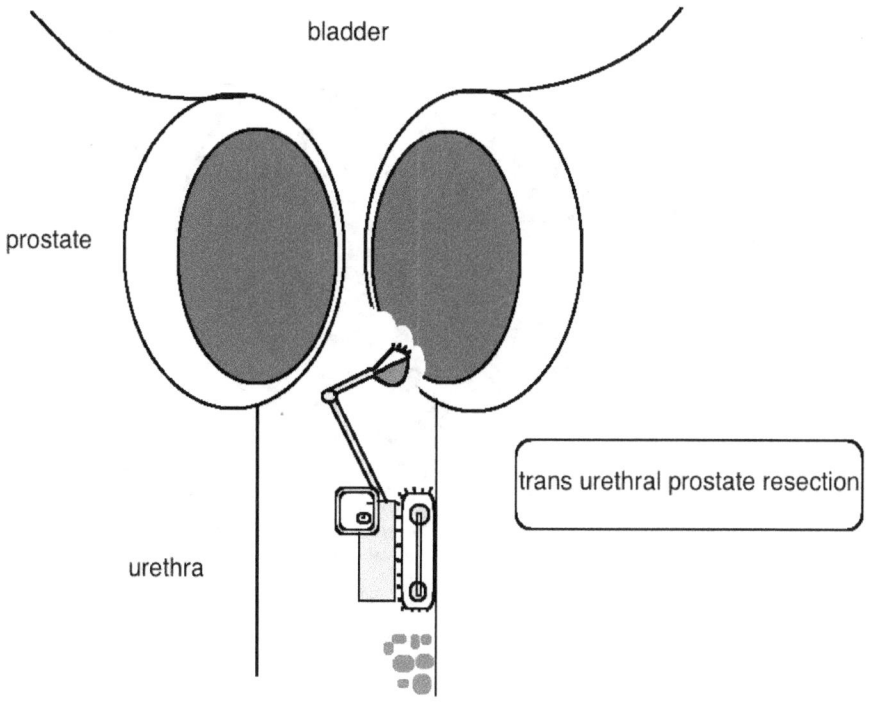

An alternative to the so-called classical resection is the **prostate laser treatment**. Its main advantage is to reduce the amount of bleeding. This technique will be particularly necessary for people with bleeding disorders, whether related to drugs (anti aggregation inhibitors, anticoagulants) or diseases (eg hemophilia).

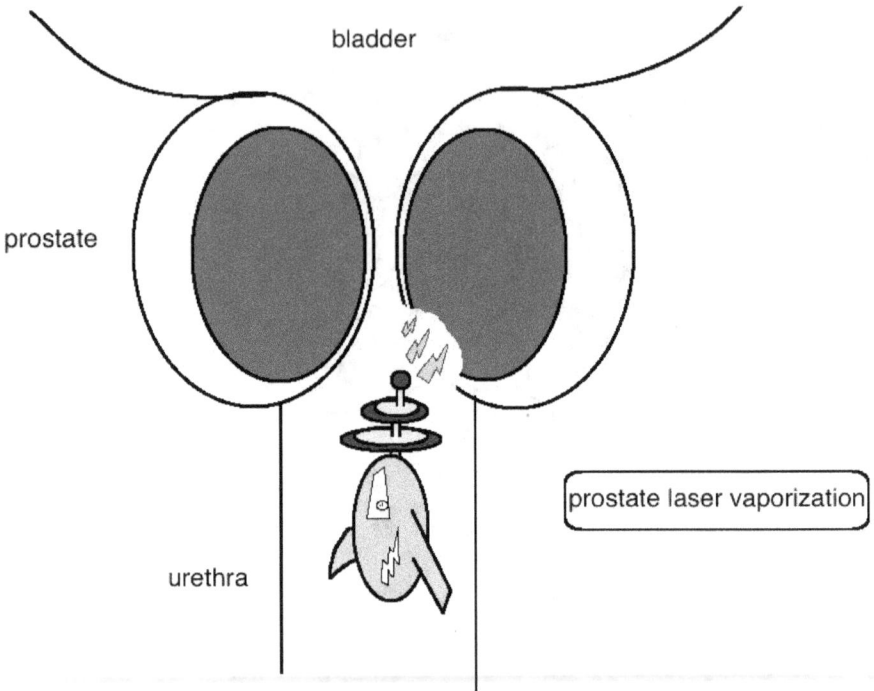

bladder

prostate

prostate laser vaporization

urethra

The thermal ablation, although less effective over time and the urine output, has the advantage of fewer complications than resection.

For very large prostates (over 90 grams), surgery incision (lower abdomen) may be preferred. This is the **open prostatectomy**.

Finally, for small prostates (under 30 gr), **bladder neck incision** will be the technique of choice. The prostate tissue is not removed but the bladder neck is broadened.

6 – ACUTE URINARY RETENTION

or sudden inability to urinate. It's very **painful**.

This blockage is often preceded by difficulty urinating in few days previous.

The causes can be many, but enlarged prostate (BPH) is the most common cause in men over 50 years. This is a **consequence of bladder outlet obstruction**.

The retention risk is particularly important when the bladder empties poorly. An ultrasound examination after urination can determine this risk by measuring the volume of urine remaining in the bladder after urination (post void volume).

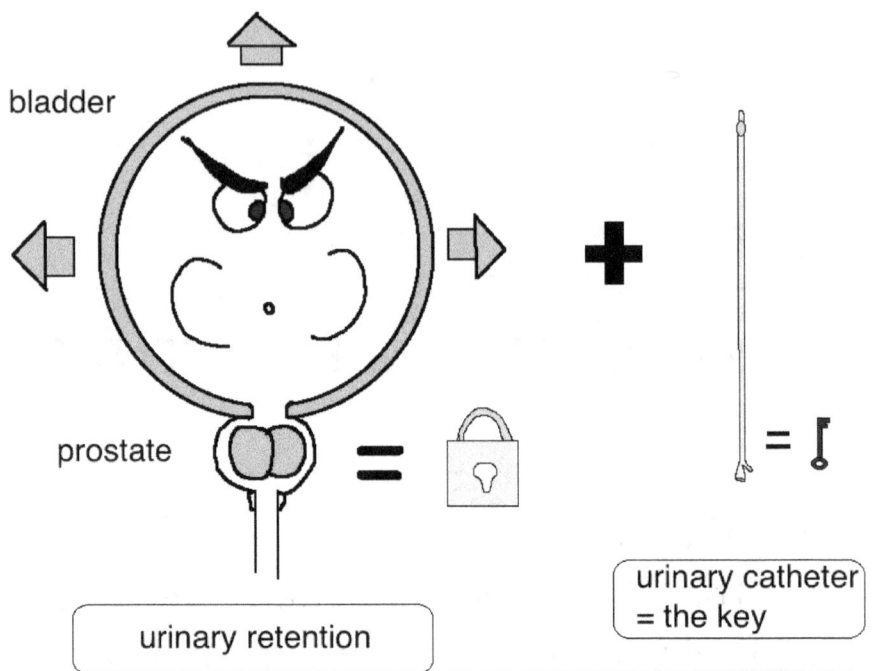

bladder

prostate

urinary retention

urinary catheter
= the key

Treatment

Bladder, although very painful, must be evacuated. A **urinary catheter** can then be implemented urgently by a doctor or nurse.

If it's not possible, or if there is a contraindication, drainage through the abdominal wall under local anesthesia is realized, that's the **suprapubic catheter.**

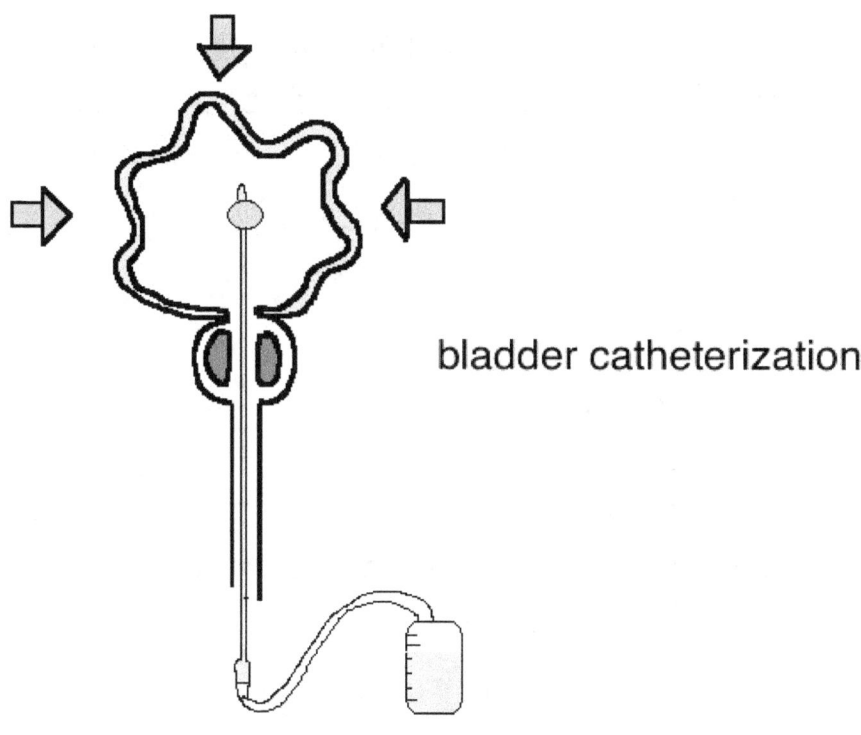

bladder catheterization

Chronic urinary retention

This situation is more dangerous because it's insidious. Indeed, the pain is not present, but bladder is full.

Urinary leakage (dribbling) occurs often called overflow incontinence, like an overfilled glass. The risk is renal insufficiency, which can lead up to dialysis.

And after...

The urinary catheter stays for several days in order allow the bladder to rest. Its removal will be followed by a good recovery urination monitoring.

This episode is often the opportunity to begin drug treatment for benign prostate hyperplasia, or if this treatment was already followed, time to suggest surgery.

7 – URINARY TRACT INFECTION IN MEN: PROSTATITIS

Prostatitis is the most frequent Urinary tract infection in men

Bacteria present in the urine come inflame the prostate. The gland then "swells" causing urinary problems: a weaker urinary flow, with frequent and painful urination. Fever and body aches are common.

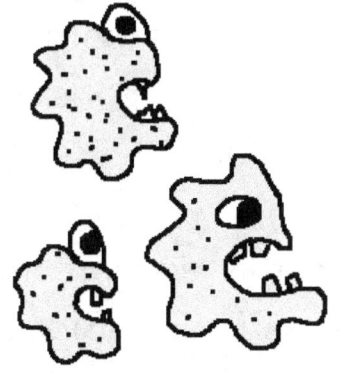 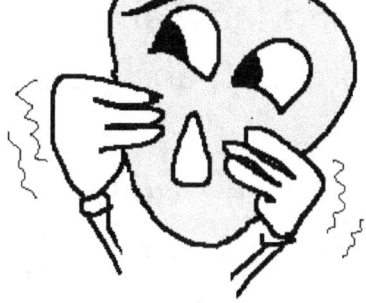

bacteria

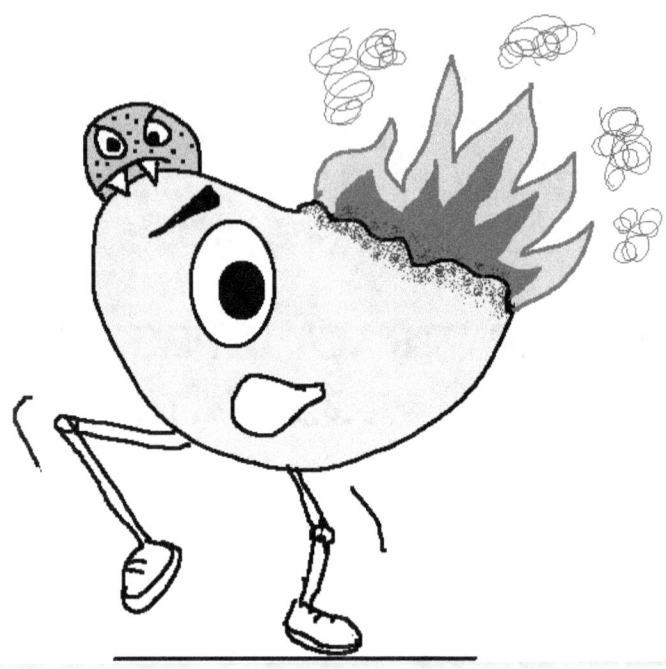

Retention of urine after 50 years is most often a complication of BPH.

The starting point is an incomplete bladder emptying. Urine is constantly present, and bacteria much like it.

The guilty bacteria in this age are from digestive origin (gut flora) as E.Coli. Blood in urine or semen, may appear.

The testis, the epididymis which covers it, or the urethra can also be the site of inflammation and infections.

Treatment

A long term antibiotic therapy of 3 to 6 weeks is required after completion of a urinalysis. Rest and painkillers are recommended.

On the same principle, drug treatment or intervention on the BPH can be offered because of the risk of recurrence.

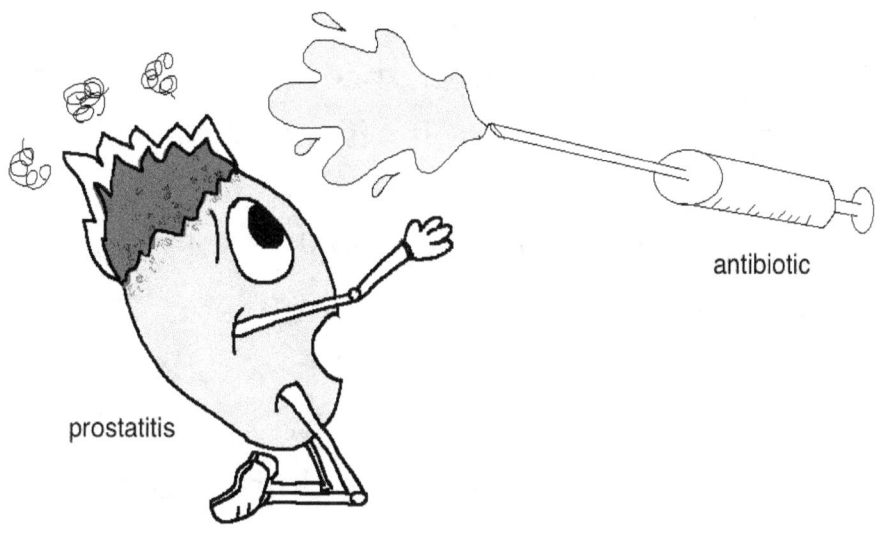

antibiotic

prostatitis

8 - PROSTATE CANCER

Prostate cancer is the most common cancer in men (10). In France around 53 500 new cases were diagnosed in 2012 and 8500 deaths. In the US, there were 220 800 new cases in 2015.

Like for all cancers, the earlier it is diagnose, the better the efficacy and so the probability to make it disappear.

Thus, the 5-year survival is 94% in France for patients diagnosed between 2005 and 2010 (11).

About 14% of men will experience a prostate cancer in the United States, one man in seven.

Risk factors

Some are known : age, heredity, that is, to have a father or brother diagnosed with prostate cancer (risk x2) or ethnicity: African American and Caribbean men being of a higher risk in contrast to Asians.

Similarly, the incidence of prostate cancer is higher in Northern Europe than in Southern Europe.

Regarding the environment, there is still unknown. If it is accepted that diet plays a role, there is to date no certainty. Studies are underway.

Exposure to chlordecone, a pesticide used in banana cultivation in the Antilles, increase the risk of prostate cancer.

If there is a risk factor, PSA testing is recommended from 45 years in Europe.

Symptoms

The whole problem is that prostate cancer shows no symptoms until an advanced stage. Contrary to what one might imagine, urinary disorders are rarely the mode of discovery of prostate cancer.

The reason is mentioned in the first chapter, urinary problems rather concern the central part of the prostate while cancer is most often at the periphery.

Finally, recent bone pains (spine, pelvis), with a context of fatigue in an aged man, need to eliminate a prostate cancer with metastasis. When the disease leaves the prostate, it will then preferentially be localized on the bones and lymph nodes.

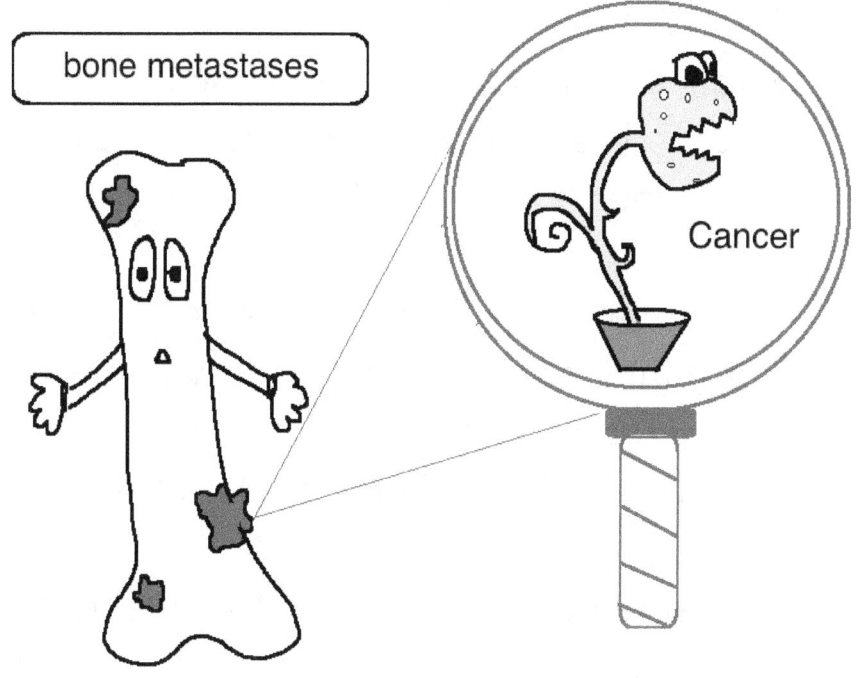

bone metastases

Cancer

Prostate cancer screening

The difficulty lies partly in the will not to ignore a severe prostatic disease for which effective treatment could be offered, and secondly not to screen and systematically treat all prostate cancer including indolent, at any price.

There are situations where the treatment and its potential consequences can be worse than the disease itself. This is the case particularly in the elderly or those with other severe diseases that life expectancy would not exceed a few years.

Currently, learned societies and Health authorities are discussing the value, interest and economical consequences of early diagnosis of prostate cancer by PSA testing.

The validated attitude to date is for an individual screening after discussion with his urologist keeping in mind existing risk factors.

The **screening tools** are the PSA, clinical examination by digital rectal examination and prostate biopsies.
We can hope that in the coming years, other ways such as prostate MRI or other biological markers will be more performant.

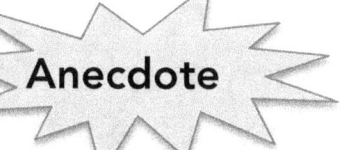

Anecdote

several studies have found evidence that specially trained dogs are capable of detecting prostate cancer in the smell of human urine; with a very impressive sensitivity (12).

Additional medical exams

In the case of prostate cancer on biopsies, some imaging exams are required in order to determine precisely the extent of the disease, the staging.

This report provides details on the size and location of the tumor, the existence of positive nodes or metastases, all summarized by **TNM stage** (Tumor Nodes Metastases).

The fundamental question at this point is: Is the disease only localized to the prostate? or Has it already spread elsewhere ?

A **bone scan** is a test performed in a Nuclear Medicine department. It studies the entire skeleton in search of bone metastases.

The **CT-scan** search anomalies in other organs, the presence of abnormal lymph nodes and provides details of the abnormalities of bone scan.

The **prostate MRI** achieves a precise examination of the local extended disease within the prostate and in its surroundings. Reading this review is difficult, made you advise a Radiologist.

Prostate cancer treatment
○ <u>Surgery</u>

<u>Prostatectomy</u>, or complete removal of the prostate, is the standard treatment for localized prostate cancer.

This procedure can be done in different ways: traditional open surgery, laparoscopic or robotic surgery.

In the latter two cases, the abdominal cavity is filled with gas to create a space for small instruments in order to move and work accurately. These instruments are introduced through small incisions. Robotic surgery in recent years is booming.

After prostatectomy, the two main problems that may be encountered are urinary incontinence (leakage), and erectile dysfunction.

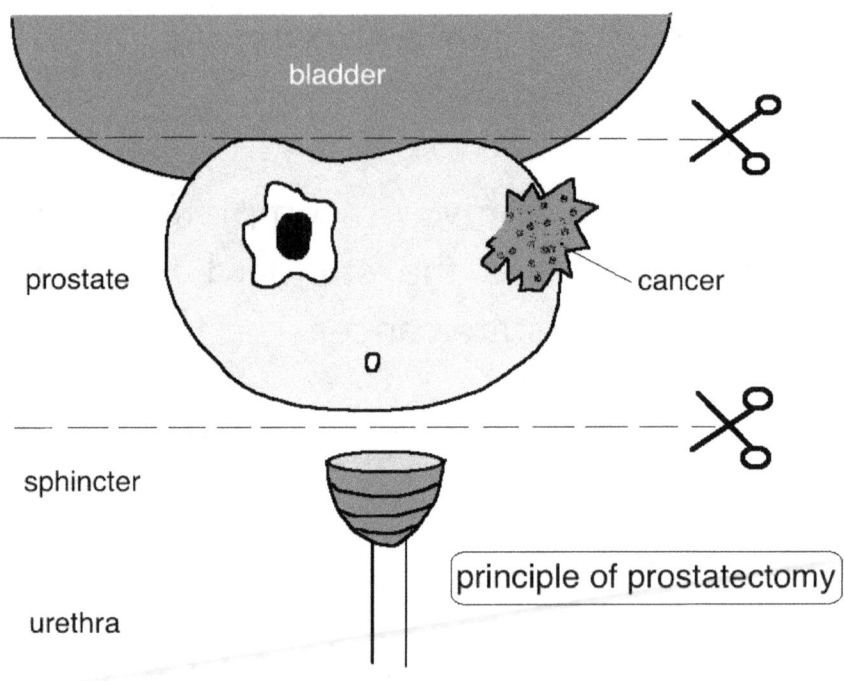

principle of prostatectomy

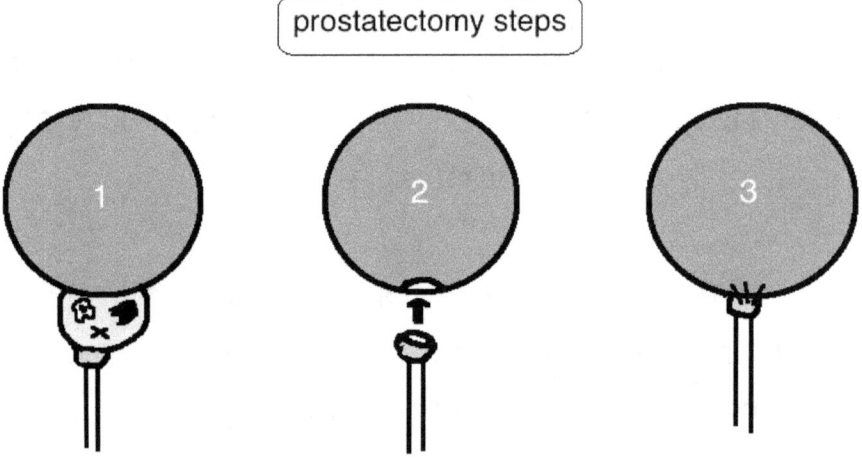

prostatectomy steps

Definitive **urinary incontinence** is rare. Recent studies estimate that nearly 84% of patients do not carry any protection one year after surgery (13). These leaks are partly explained by the proximity of the striated sphincter of the urethra and prostate. This sphincter is somewhat like a tap that can be closed to refrain from urinating.

In case of persistent urinary leakage, solutions exist, including surgical interventions that allow a significant improvement (ex : artificial urinary sphincter).

urinary stress incontinence

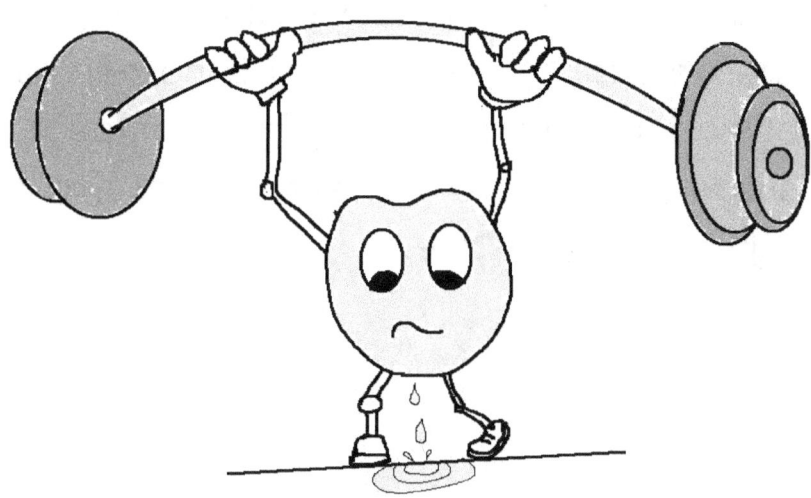

<u>Sexual dysfunction</u> after prostate removal are unfortunately more common.

First, there 's no more ejaculation because seminal vesicles are removed during the procedure.

On the other hand, although many will return erections, it is estimated that approximately 25% of patients become naturally erect for satisfactory sexual intercourse (without drugs) (14).

Depending on the characteristics of cancer determind by various examinations, the decision to retain or not the nerves that allow for erection, is in general made before surgery. These nerves are fragile and glued against the prostate.

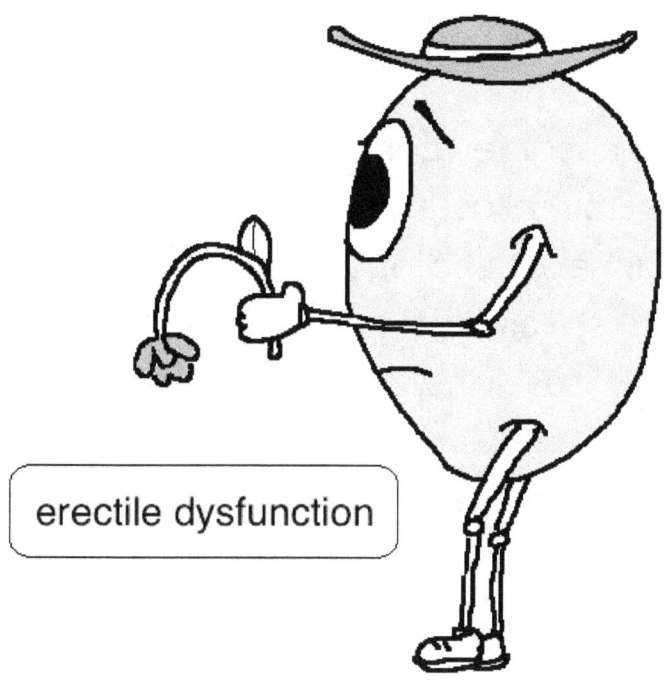

erectile dysfunction

When the decision is to keep them, the difficulty is not to get too close to the affected area.

Apart from this nerve preservation, the results on the ability to regain erections depend on preoperative criteria such as age, quality of erections before surgery, the presence of other associated health problems, but also after treatment, the couple motivation (15).

o <u>Radiotherapy</u>

A machine containing a power source sends ray prostate to destroy cancer cells. The dose of radioactivity to be delivered is "split" so as not to be toxic. This involves many sessions, 4-5 per week for approximately 6 weeks. Several protocols exist that can vary these durations.

The side effects encountered are mainly inflammation of the bladder or rectum. The symptoms are frequent desire, even urgent, to urinate. This can happen in a short period during treatment, or more definitively after several years. Bleeding in the urine or stool may also occur over time.

On a sexual note, half or two-thirds of patients will gradually become impotent after a few years (16).

○ <u>Brachytherapy</u>

This treatment is also based on the radioactivity, but this time the power source is internal, in the prostate.

Tiny radioactive seeds are placed in the prostate, under anesthesia. These grains, also called implants can be temporary or permanent. In the latter case, the radioactivity is exhausted with time to become almost zero.

Brachytherapy cannot be performed on large prostate or when the patient suffers from important urinary disorders, or if a previous trans urethral resection of the prostate was realized.

Side effects are also primarily related to inflammation or bleeding of the bladder and rectum. Persistant bladder irritation continues in 10% of cases.

o <u>Ultrasounds</u>

High intensity focused ultrasound treatment is being evaluated. An endo-rectal probe should be in place during treatment.

Currently this technique is preferentially offered to patient older than 70 patients or younger patients if they have other severe diseases.

Adverse effects, urinary incontinence is seen in almost a third of cases, and a narrowing of the urethra or bladder neck in 17% of cases.

o <u>Cryotherapy</u>

Also being evaluated, rather reserved for small prostates. This treatment is by cold, under anesthesia. Erection disorders are common after treatment in 50-90% of cases.

o <u>Hormonotherapy</u>

This is the standard treatment for **metastatic prostate cancer**.

Its use in localized cancers is possible, in combination with radiotherapy.

The principle is based on castration. Indeed, the goal of these drugs is to reduce to the lowest testosterone production. This hormone is the "fuel" of prostate cancer, and 90% of it is produced by the testes. Either an intervention removes the testicles or their content, (but this is rarely done nowadays), or a treatment is administred.

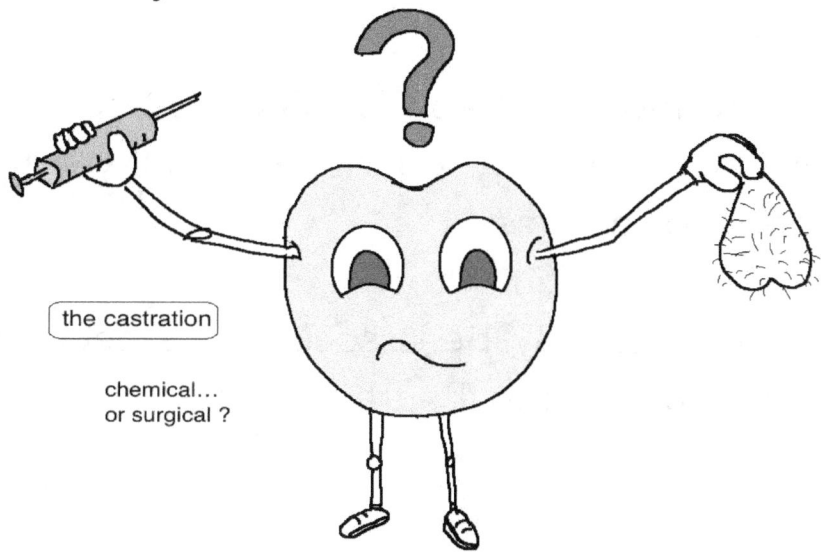

the castration

chemical...
or surgical ?

The Hormone therapy will not be able to remove the cancer, but it will try to block it.

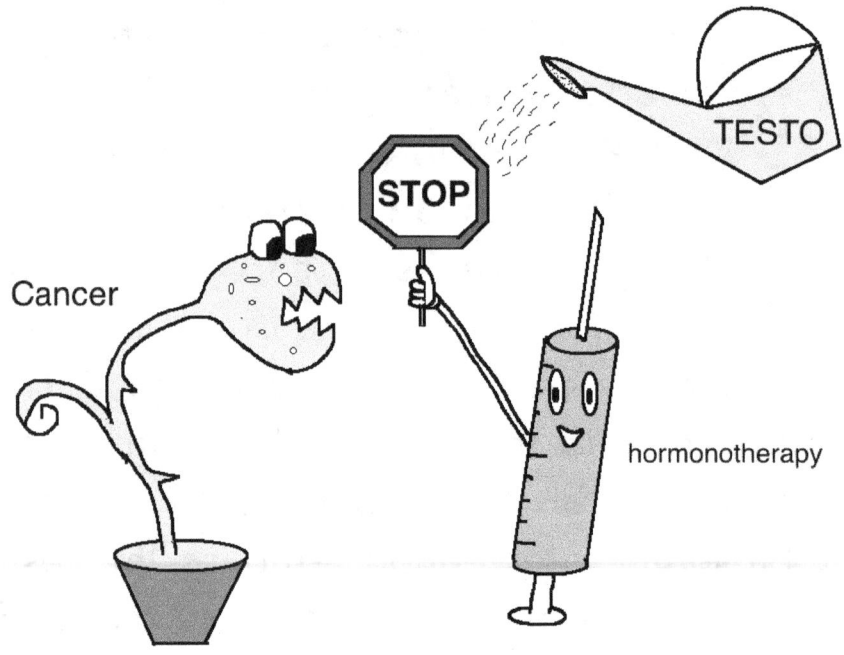

Hormone therapy is mainly based on an injection, monthly, quarterly, or half-yearly, at home by a nurse.

Tablets may be associated, especially in the beginning of the treatment.

Overall, this treatment is well tolerated. The main side effects are hot flashes, decreased libido and erections, slight weight gain, possibly some mood disorders, etc...

The duration of treatment efficacy is limited in time. The disease becomes resistant after a variable time. Other drugs can then be prescribed : "new" hormones therapies or chemotherapy.

9 – LIFESTYLE AND PROSTATE

Here is a list of foods that are likely to play a role in the onset or progression of prostate cancer (17) :

These foods would help to reduce the risk of prostate cancer

- Soy and its derivatives (isoflavones)
- Cabbage, broccoli, cauliflower (iso thiocyanate)
- Garlic, onions, shallots
- Vitamin C (peppers, broccoli, cabbage, citrus)
- Vitamin K (spinach, broccoli)
- Coffee

These foods would increase the risk of prostate cancer

- Red meat (well cooked)
- Dairy products (saturated fats and calcium)
- Polyunsaturated omega 6
- Excessive vitamin supplementation (vitamin E)

These foods would slow the prostate cancer growth

- Oily fish (tuna, trout, salmon, mackerel, etc.): rich in Omega 3
- Linseed
- Vitamin C (antioxidant)
- Vitamin E (corn oil, sunflower, palm) (antioxidant)
- Curcumin
- Pomegranate
- Nuts

- Green tea (antioxidant)
- Tomatoes, cooked or sauce, watermelon and grapes (lycopene)

On vitamin D and selenium, contrary to what has often been read, the studies do not appear to show a clear association between these products and the risk of prostate cancer (18, 19).

All is in the dose

Paracelsus, a doctor of the sixteenth century said " All things are poisons, for there is nothing without poisonous qualities. It is only the dose which makes a thing poison"

Here is the illustration of those substances considered to be protective against cancer. A good example is vitamin E whose daily recommendation is estimated to be 15 mg after 50 years. It is found in sunflower oil, avocado, nuts, almonds, etc ...

Studies have shown that a normal dose could slow the progression of prostate cancer, but high doses of vit. E in dietary supplements can increase the risk of prostate cancer (20).

The same can be said for polyunsaturated fatty acids Omega 3, they could help reduce the development of prostate cancer in normal doses, but again, taken in high quantities, they would have the opposite effect (21).

Physical activity

Physical activity is associated with a slightly decreased risk of prostate cancer (22).

Obesity appears to be linked to forms of more aggressive prostate cancer and with PSA levels lower, it is less likely to be diagnosed.

Tobacco

Smokers would be at higher risk of cancer recurrence for patient who were treated by surgery (prostatectomy) (23).

What conclusions ?

Finally, The Mediterranean diet probably includes most foods which protect against the prostate cancer risk and its progression.

Moreover, the Mediterranean diet is associated with a decreased risk of cancer in general and coronary heart disease.

Countries practicing this diet have lower incidence and mortality linked on prostate cancer (24).

The Mediterranean diet

It is known to be composed of many fruits and vegetables, olive oil, cereals, fish, with moderate alcohol consumption (especially wine), low consumption of milk and dairy products as well as meats (particularly red).

Another conclusion from these studies, it is distrusting of these **food supplements** promising protection against prostate cancer. These products generally have not been studied.

10 – SEXUALITY AND PROSTATE

The only real recognized role of the prostate is to help in the process of ejaculation.

On this occasion, the prostate and seminal vesicles contract to expel the semen into the urethra, all under neurological control.

The increase in prostate volume with age can disrupt the functioning of sexuality via erectile dysfunction and premature ejaculation. One study showed that 88% of men 50 to 80 years old had ejaculation disorders (25).

More urinary problems are severe therfore the frequency of sexual activity would be reduced (26).

The treatment of benign prostatic hyperplasia, whether medical or surgical, can in turn cause these same sexual disorders. For example with **retrograde ejaculation**, which consists of expulsion seminal fluid in the wrong direction, ie into the bladder rather than out. This presents no danger or pain, but can be frustrating for some very savvy men.

In prostatitis, ejaculation may be painful or colored red / brown because semen contains blood.

On prostate cancer, the disease development in itself beyond the prostate may have an impact on erections.

As we saw in a previous chapter, all

prostate cancer treatments affect sexuality, even apart from the psychological impact associated with the disease. Most often it is the nerves of erection that are harmed because of their proximity from the prostate.

Another mechanism is the drop in libido when testosterone collapses during treatment with hormone therapy.

Even patients in Active surveillance would have a progressive deterioration of their sexuality during the first two years, independantly with the number of biopsies or patient anxiety, but it would mitigate with time (27).

Fortunately, more and more treatments appear for erectile dysfunction in different forms: tablets, gels, injections to the penis, not to mention the vacuum pump and penile prostheses .

A word from the author

At a time when the web offers us an infinite source of information but uncontrolled, the goal here is to provide simple answers to patient's questions by providing a reliable source, based on international guidelines, but also to clear up some preconceptions.

REFERENCES

1- Catalona et al . Mesurement of prostate specific antigen in serum as a screening test for prostatic cancer. New England Journal of Medecine 1991 ; 324 :1156-1161

2- Greene et al. Prostate specific antigen best practice statement : 2009 update. Journal of Urology 2013 ;105 :52-511

3- Andriole et al. Effects of dutasteride on the risk of prostate cancer. New Englan Journal of Medecine 2010 April : 362(13) :1192-202

4- Leibovitch et al. The Vicious Cycling: Bicycling Related Urogenital Disorders . European Urology 47 (2005) 277–287

5- Richie et al. Effect of patient age on early detection of prostate cancer with serum prostate specific antigen and digital rectal examination. Urology 1993 oct 42(4) :365-74

6- B . Van Asseldouk et al. Medical therapy for benigne prostatic hyperplasia : a review. The Canadian Journal of

Urology 2015 ;22 :7-17

7- Kristal et al. Race, ethnicity, obesity, health related behaviors and the risk of symptomatic benign prostatic hyperplasia: result from the prostate cancer prevention trial. Journal of Urology 2007 ; 177

8- Habib et al. Not all brands are created equal : a comparison of selected components of different brands of Serenoa repens extract. Prostate Cancer Prostatic Disease 2004 ; 7(3) :195-200

9- Williams et al. A high ratio of dietary n-6/n-3 poly insaturated fat acids is associated with increased risk of prostate cancer. Nutrition Research 2011

10-Binder-Foucard et al. Cancer incidence and mortality in France over the 1980-2012 period: solid tumors. Rev Epidemiol Sante Publique 2014;62(2):95-108

11 - Survie des personnes atteintes de cancer en France métropolitaine, 1989-2013. Partie 1 – Tumeurs solides. Institut de veille sanitaire. 2016

12- Cornu et al. Olfactory detection of prostate cancer by dogs sniffing urine : a step forward in early diagnosis. European Urology. 2011 february ;59 :197-201

13- Ficarra et al. Systematic review and meta analysis of studies reporting urinary incontinence recovery after robot assisted radical prostatectomy. European Urology 2012 ;

62 :405-17

14- Ficarra et al. Systematic review and meta analysis of studies reporting potency rates after robot assisted radical prostatectomy. European Urology 2012 ;62 :418-30

15- Pumeur et al. Long term health related quality of life after primary treatment for localized prostate cancer : results from the CAPSURE registry. European Urology 2014

16- www.e-cancer.fr site de l'institut national du cancer

17- Masko et al. The Relationship Between Nutrition and Prostate Cancer: Is More Always Better? European Uroloy 2013 ;63 :810-820

18- Klein et al. Vitamin E and the risk of prostate cancer: the Selenium and Vitamin E Cancer Prevention Trial (SELECT). JAMA 2011;306:1549–56.

19- Gilbert et al. Associations of circulating and dietary vitamin D with prostate cancer risk: a systematic review and dose-response meta-analysis. Cancer Causes Control 2011;22:319–40.

20- Klein et al. Vitamine E and the risk of prostate cancer : the selenium and vitamine E cancer prevention trial (SELECT). JAMA 2011 ;306 :1549-56

21- Brasky et al. Plasma phospholipid fatty acid and prostate cncer risk. J Natl Cancer Inst 2013;105:1132–41

22- Yu Peng Liu et al. Does physical activity reduce the risk of prostate cancer ? a systematic review and meta analysis. European Urology 2011 ;60 :1120-1124

23- Rieken et al. Association of Cigarette Smoking and Smoking Cessation with Biochemical Recurrence of Prostate Cancer in Patients Treated with Radical Prostatectomy. European Urology 2015 ;68 :949-956

24- Kenfield et al. Mediterranean diet and prostate cancer risk and mortality in the health professionals follow up study. European Urology 2014 ;65 :887-894

25- Rosen et al. Lower urinary tract symptoms and male sexual dysfunction : te multinational survey of the aging male (MSAM-7). European Urology 2003 ;44 :637-645

26- Colson et al. Conséquences psychologiques et sexuelles de l'hypertrophie bénigne de prostate. Sexologies 2014 ;23 :85-90

27- Pearce et al. A Longitudinal Study of Predictors of Sexual Dysfunction in Men on Active Surveillance for Prostate Cancer. Sexual Medicine 2015;3:156–164

THE AUTHOR :

Dr. Bertrand Vayleux is Urologist.

He realized his medical studies in France.

He exercises in the South West of France.